The Learning About Myself (LAMS) Program for At-Risk Parents
Handbook for Group Participants

The Learning About Myself (LAMS) Program for At-Risk Parents
Handbook for Group Participants

Verna Rickard, BSW, LSW

HMTP

The Haworth Maltreatment and Trauma Press
An Imprint of The Haworth Press, Inc.

Published by

The Haworth Maltreatment and Trauma Press, an imprint of The Haworth Press, Inc., 10 Alice Street, Binghamton, NY 13904-1580

Cover design by Monica L. Seifert.

Library of Congress Cataloging-in-Publication Data

Rickard, Verna.
  The learning about myself (LAMS) program for at-risk parents : Handbook for group participants / Verna Rickard.
      p.   cm.
  Includes bibliographical references and index.
  ISBN 0-7890-0471-2 (alk. paper).
  1. Social group work 2. Self-actualization (Psychology). I. Title.
HV45.R515 1998
361.4—dc21   97-45067
                                                                                                          CIP

CONTENTS

You can learn to change your life
by choosing so to do,
What you were and who you were
can now be something new.

About Your Book

In LAMS group you will learn many things but will have fun along the way. When you have completed the program, you should feel better about yourself and your life. LAMS will help you understand how what happened to you in the past affects how you feel about yourself now. It will also teach you some basic skills to help you live the best life possible. You will discover how you make choices; learn how to set goals; get along with others; look and feel better; and even how to feed your family a balanced diet.

This is your handbook. You will be using it in group every week. It is divided into weekly sections, one for each of the fifteen weeks of the LAMS course. When you arrive each week, turn to the section for the week and topic being covered. You will read the affirmation aloud, together with the leaders and other group members. There may be other readings for the week; the leader will read them, but you can follow along in your book.

Sometimes there are special activities or questions in your handbook, and you should take notes about things you learn. This is *your* book, and the things you add are things that mean something to you. You will also play games every week, but those are not listed in your book; the leaders will tell you what to do.

Every weekly section has a page or two that tells you what will be covered in that session, and in a few sections, there are several pages that explain things in more detail. When you complete all fifteen weeks of the LAMS program, or if you have to leave for some reason, you will keep your handbook. You can use it to help you remember the things you learned in LAMS, and you may want to share parts of it with others in your family.

The LAMS program will help you learn from the past and give you the information you need to change your future. If you really want to change your life, you can, and LAMS can help—but nobody can *make* you change—you have to *want* things to be different. This handbook is your key to open the door to a better life.

Week One: My Self

Your brain is almost like a computer. It stores everything that happens to you from the time you are born. When you make choices, you remember things from many parts of your brain, things you may not even know you know are there. You make choices thousands of times every day; most of them you do not even think about. You remember how to walk, how to eat, and how to find places you want to go. You learned a long time ago that if you drop something, it might break; if you skip school, you might get caught; and if you steal, you might go to jail. The choices you make are based on all of the things you have learned in your lifetime. When needed, your brain decides in only seconds what choice you are going to make.

If you make the wrong choice, you will have to live with what happens to you, but you *make* a choice; life does not just *happen* to you. You are the one who can change your life by the choices you make; you are the one who is in control. You can live your life by *choice*, not by *chance*.

AFFIRMATION

I am important.
What I say is important.
What I think is important.
What I do is important,
To myself and those around me.
I choose to be the best, most caring, accepting,
    and understanding person I can be.

MAKING CHOICES

You may feel that a lot of things have just "happened" to you in your life. Really, *you* have made them happen. Your past choices have put you where you are today.

When you learn how to make the right choices, you can choose what you want your life to be like and change what it is like now.

You can choose to live your life by *choice*, not by *chance*.

I'M OK

I'm really OK. I will learn to like myself. I will do nice things for myself, or by myself. I will treat myself to things I really want to do, such as read a book or go for a walk. I don't have to do what other people want me to do all of the time. I am still "me" inside, even if I am a mother or father, a child to my own parents, a wife or girlfriend, or a husband or boyfriend. I have needs of my own, and time I spend alone helps me to understand who I am. I do not have to like everybody, and everybody does not have to like me. I will change myself, even though I cannot change others. I will say good things to myself and tell myself I am a good person. This may be hard because I don't always feel like those things are true. I will think about what I *can* do, not what I *cannot* do. I will be good to my body by eating right and taking care of myself, so I will feel better and look better. I will be nice to others and say nice things to them so they will like themselves better, too. I will enjoy being the great person that I am!

CHOICES QUESTIONNAIRE

These questions are to help you learn about yourself and do not have to be handed in.

1. Is your life better than your mother's or father's was?

   Yes _____ No _____ Undecided _____

2. Do you think your life will be better five years from now?

   Yes _____ No _____ Undecided _____

3. Do you think your children will have a better life than you have had?

   Yes _____ No _____ Undecided _____

4. Would your life be different today if you had:

Different parents?	Y_____	N_____	U_____
More education?	Y_____	N_____	U_____
Gotten involved with someone else?	Y_____	N_____	U_____
Not had children at a young age?	Y_____	N_____	U_____
More money?	Y_____	N_____	U_____

5. Has your life changed through:

Decisions *you* made?	Y_____	N_____	U_____
Decisions *others* made for you?	Y_____	N_____	U_____
Things that just happened?	Y_____	N_____	U_____

6. Most of the time, are you doing what:

You want to do?	Y_____	N_____	U_____
Others want you to do?	Y_____	N_____	U_____

7. Have you ever had a substance abuse
problem?   Y____ N____ U____

8. Do you think women have more
self-control than men?   Y____ N____ U____

9. Do you believe you can change the
person you have a relationship with?   Y____ N____ U____

10. Do you have to have a man/woman
in your life to be happy?   Y____ N____ U____

11. What things do you do to get your own way in a disagree-
ment with your mate?

Check all that apply:

Argue   ____

Reason   ____

Pout   ____

Withhold sex   ____

Trick him or her   ____

Threaten to leave   ____

12. Not counting regular bills or expenses, how much money
would you spend without talking it over with your mate?

$10-$20   ____

$20-$50   ____

$50-$100   ____

More?   ____

13. Which of these things do you usually do for your mate?

Buy clothing?   ____

Wash clothing?   ____

Iron or put away clothing? ＿＿＿

Cook meals? ＿＿＿

Entertain his or her family or friends? ＿＿＿

Wait on him or her? ＿＿＿

Make medical or other appointments? ＿＿＿

14. How well could your mate get along without you:

    For everyday needs? Very well ＿＿ OK ＿＿ Not at all ＿＿

    Emotionally? ＿＿ ＿＿ ＿＿

    Financially? ＿＿ ＿＿ ＿＿

    Sexually? ＿＿ ＿＿ ＿＿

15. How well could your family manage without you for a few days?

    Very well ＿＿ OK ＿＿ Not at all ＿＿

16. How would you feel if they did well without you for that time?

    Awful, not needed ＿＿ OK ＿＿ Makes no difference ＿＿

17. Who decides:

    What you watch on TV? You ＿＿ Mate ＿＿ Kid ＿＿

    What is for dinner? ＿＿ ＿＿ ＿＿

    Who your friends are? ＿＿ ＿＿ ＿＿

18. How often do your needs come before those of your family?

    Sometimes ＿＿ Always ＿＿ Never ＿＿

19. Do you think men and women have equal opportunities:

    At work? Yes ＿＿No ＿＿

    At home? ＿＿ ＿＿

20. If you don't work now, would you go to work if you could get affordable daycare?

    Yes _____ No _____

21. Do you sometimes do things yourself because you feel only you can do things the right way?

    Yes _____ No _____

22. Do you sometimes feel that life just "happens" to you and you have no control?

    Yes _____ No _____

23. Do you feel that you have more problems than most people?

    Yes _____ No _____

24. Check one—Would you say that your life is generally:

    The best?   _____
    Better than most?   _____
    About average?   _____
    Worse than most?   _____
    The pits?   _____

HOW YOU MAKE CHOICES

Brain and Computer

Your brain is similar to a computer. Computers store large quantities of information and keep all of that information in order. Your brain does the same thing. Everything that is fed into a computer is registered there, regardless of whether it is put in yesterday, today, or tomorrow. Computers don't "forget" things, even though what they know may not be on the screen and available to be read all the time. The same thing happens with your memory. Everything is there. Sometimes you may have covered something up so you don't *have* to remember it, but it is still there somewhere. The main difference is that something can be erased from a computer but not from your brain, except possibly from some accidentally caused brain damage. All that information can be called up at any time.

Here is a picture of a big, four-drawer file cabinet. In the top drawer are all the new skills you learned as a baby, such as how to eat and drink, how to crawl, and even how to walk. Some other examples are how to recognize Mom, Dad, and other caretakers, know and respond to your own name, and identify animals and the sounds they make. Since you have grown up, you do not have to tell your body how to walk across the room. At one time, when you were first learning to walk, you had to think about how to hold your body, how to move your legs and feet, and how to keep your balance. Now you eat without thinking, talk easily, and get through your day with little thought to those basic skills. They are all easier, but only after a lot of practice.

Later on, you made another file in your brain to hold what you learned in your preschool years. In that drawer, you filed away how to go to the bathroom instead of wearing diapers, how to play with other children, how to tie your shoes, how to identify what you saw in your world, how to say "no" and be your own person, and millions of other pieces of information you needed to live your life.

The third drawer contains what you learned in school, such as how to read and write. What else did you learn in school? You used those basic skills as building blocks to learn more about your world.

In the fourth drawer, you stored away all of your other experiences—what happened to you before, while, or since you were in school. These might include your reactions to what people said to you, whether good or bad. This drawer would contain your opinions and ideas, your hopes and fears, and how you feel about yourself now. It would include your prejudices and what you think is right or wrong.

Of course your brain is much more complicated than a computer; this is only an example. You do not really have file cabinets to store the information, but it *is* all there someplace, filed away even when you aren't using it. Every time you make a decision or a choice, you get information out of one or more, and maybe even *all* of those drawers. Your life is not just "happening" to you; you are *choosing* your own path.

Think about how you make decisions. You make them all day, every day. Your first choice of the day may be how quickly you get up when the alarm goes off or when you wake up and know you have to get out of bed. Do you push the "snooze" button or close your eyes for "just another minute" of sleep? Look back at those file drawers. How do you know how to reach for the clock? How do you know what the "snooze" button is or what it is for? Why do you feel that you must have another minute of sleep? Did your mother let you stay in bed for a while after she first called you, and were you sure she would come back and call you again? Is there somebody with you now that you are sure will wake you up if you go back to sleep? Look in the last drawer— the one with your beliefs and ideas in it. If you don't get your kids off to school, will you hear your mother in your head telling you that you are a poor parent and a bad person? Will you feel you are not being responsible if you do not get to your doctor appointment or to work? Or did your caretakers skip such obligations regularly when you were a child? How did you learn to tell time in the first place?

As you can see, those file drawers and that computer in your head can have a big influence on how you act today and on what choices you make for yourself. You, alone, are not making those choices; in fact—much of the time—you do not even recognize that they *are* choices.

Now we will go on to a more difficult choice. Suppose you need money for groceries to feed your children. You are not due to get any money for at least a week. What kind of decisions could you make, and why would you make them?

Your first choice might be not to buy groceries at all. Why would you do that? You and your family are hungry, but you can borrow or beg some food from family or friends. How you feel about those people, and how they feel about you, might affect that choice. Maybe you have run out of food before and asked your family for help, and you remember that they said they would not help you again. Maybe you have asked the neighbors for help many times, also. You may also have too much pride (remembered from your files) to ask anyone for help even if you think they might help.

Now think of other possible ways to get money. You do not have a job, so that is not a choice. If you could get a job, you would not get money right away. Maybe you could *steal* some money? Now you get input from your files again. How do you feel about stealing? Do you feel it is wrong? (moral teaching, maybe from church as a child). Do you only fear getting caught by the police? (maybe from knowing someone who got arrested). How did your parents feel about stealing? (maybe they did it all the time, or maybe they would have never stolen for any reason). Would you be embarrassed if your friends found out you stole something? After considering everything in your file drawers, your choice is made in seconds. We never think about the memories behind the choices we make, any more than we think about what we have to do to walk across the room.

Your final choice made, in order to get food, may be to go to the nearest church that you know has a free food program, tell them what your problem is, and get help there. That is morally okay; you will not get arrested or be embarrassed in front of your friends; your parents will not be unhappy with you, and your children will get food.

That choice takes information out of many of your file drawers. You have to know how to get to the church, what days they give out food, what time of day to go, how to read the name of the church, and how to fill out the application form. Maybe you had to call the church first, before you went, to find out what you needed to know. After you get the food, you have to know how to get back home, how to prepare it, and even how to pick up the fork or spoon to get it into your mouth. And you thought making choices was *simple*!

Can any of you think of some examples of choices you have made already today? From now on, do not make all of your choices without thinking about them. What you buy at the grocery store is a choice. You can spend all of your money on junk food and be out of money by next week, or you can choose to shop sensibly, buy things that stretch your money, and have some left at the end of the month. That is a *choice;* it does not just *happen.* If you do not pay the rent, you are *choosing* to possibly be evicted. If you do not want to be evicted, you would have to make a different choice, such as going to get help, trying to work something out with your landlord, getting help from a friend, or moving somewhere else you could afford. Life does not just *happen* to you; the choices you make are your own, and life just follows along. If you take drugs, you may become an addict. If you drink heavily, you will probably get drunk. Everything you do has a result, or a consequence, and if you think about those consequences *before* you make your choices, your life will be in *your* control.

This is what you will be learning in LAMS every week—how you can be in charge of your life. Many of you did not learn how to do this at home; some of you may not have thought it was *possible* to be in control. Some people say they cannot do it because of what happened to them as children, or because everyone dislikes them, or they do not have much education, or they are only twenty-one years old and have three children. These are just excuses—you *can* learn to be in charge; in fact, you have already learned today how and why you make the choices you make and how to put more thought into them. You have learned that nothing "out there" controls you—you do it yourself.

Week Two: My Attitude

The little voice in your head, your "self-talk," needs to tell you that you are a good person. If it does, you feel good about yourself and what kind of person you are. If all you hear are hurtful words you will feel like you are a bad person. How you think controls how you feel.

If what you hear in your head is always bad, you need to change that to positive thoughts. You may have heard mean, hurtful statements from others when you were little, and you still may think they are true. Tell yourself you are able to accomplish whatever you try, that you are smart, that you deserve to be loved, that you *can* do what you want to do. Changing what that voice says is hard, but with practice, it can be done.

Learn to be yourself, not somebody who has to do what other people want you to do all of the time. You have your own thoughts and feelings; you are a person with rights, and you are special. If your attitude is positive, it will rub off on other people. Be somebody other people want to be around because you make them feel good about you and about themselves.

AFFIRMATION

I choose to have a good attitude.
I will see life as good.
I will be myself and not hide behind a mask.
I will do everything I can to see the best in myself
    and others around me.

ATTITUDE IS CONTAGIOUS

Have you ever had a *really* bad day—one when everything you did was wrong? It all started when you kicked the edge of the door on the way to the bathroom; what you wanted to wear was dirty; and the hot water was cold. By the time you got to the kitchen you were cross and out of sorts. Your children made you angry because they were slow getting to the table for breakfast. Your husband could not find what he needed for work, and you were *not* in the mood to help him look for it. The school bus was early, and the kids were late. Your good-bye as they went out the door was angry and frustrated.

What about *their* day? How did your attitude affect them? Probably they were short-tempered with their friends, sarcastic when answering their teachers, and spoiling for an argument until later in the day, when the effects of your mood wore off.

Now think of the opposite. What about a *great* day? You bounced out of bed, the sun was shining, and you looked forward to your trip to the store. You complimented your teenaged daughter on her choice of clothing, telling her how nice she looked. You told your son he had done a really good job cleaning up the yard, and let your husband know you especially liked his new tie. All the family responded to your good mood, being positive themselves. You smiled at the kids when they left for school and told them you loved them.

What about the rest of their day? Exactly. *Your* attitude changed *their* attitude. They gave compliments to their friends, were pleasant to their teachers, and were nicer to everyone they met.

Remember that "glow" you feel for hours after someone tells you how nice you look or how pretty your shirt is? What about the opposite—when the checker at the grocery store is rude and disagreeable? You often respond in the same manner. We all need to remember that it costs nothing extra to be kind and polite to others, and hopefully, they will pass it on to everyone they meet later in the day. Not only colds are contagious—attitude is too!

THE POWER OF THOUGHT

Have you ever heard a little voice in your head talking to you? . . . No, I do not mean that I think you are crazy. I am talking about the voice that says, "Stupid, why did you say that? You never can keep your mouth shut!" or "There you go again, always making mistakes." That little voice is called "self-talk." Your mind does it even while your body is doing something else. If what you hear in your head is positive—telling you that you are a good person—you probably feel good about yourself. If all you hear is that you are bad, you probably feel depressed and down. How you *think* controls how you *feel.*

Think about how you talk to yourself. Would you say those hurtful words to a friend? If not, how can you learn to love yourself and forgive yourself for making mistakes? . . . (Tell yourself you are a great person.)

We begin each LAMS session with an Affirmation, something to help you focus on good things you can tell yourself. Listen to what you hear in your head. If your little voice never says anything good, teach it something new. If you always hear that you are "stupid," stop and think where that came from. Did your parents say that, and did you think it was true then? Is it true *now*? If not, tell yourself you are smart, and you can learn to do anything. Until you *think* you can, you *cannot.* Changing what that little voice says is hard, but with practice you can do it.

Week Three: My Relationships

Do you live your life bending and twisting to please others? Do your needs and wants come last, behind those of your husband or boyfriend or wife or girlfriend and your kids? You have a right to be your own person; you do not have to be a slave for your family. You do not "deserve" to be abused by anyone, no matter what you do or do not do. You will never get the respect you deserve unless you ask for it.

You do not have to please other people all of the time. You do not have to feel guilty for wanting something for yourself once in a while. You can learn to be assertive and tell people what you want and need and not continue to live your life doing what everyone else wants.

AFFIRMATION

I choose to talk in a way that tells others what
    I am thinking and allows them to see the best in me.
I choose to believe in others and help them
    to believe in themselves.
I will appreciate others for who they are
    and not try to change them.
I will learn to control my temper and treat others fairly.
I will listen to others and consider their opinions,
But I will choose to do what is right for *me*.

DO YOU HAVE TO PLEASE?

Are you a "pretzel" person? Are you somebody who has to bend and twist to please others? Many people, women especially, were raised to believe that they need to please everyone. Do you put your needs or wants after your husband's or boyfriend's and your children's?

Years ago women seldom worked away from home. They were expected to take care of the children and have food on the table at mealtimes. They may have eaten only after everyone else was served. They were considered as almost second-class citizens. Men were the important people in the world. That is where the "pleaser" idea came from—the role that women were expected to fill.

Today women's roles have changed. Women are doctors, pilots, lawyers, and leaders in business and government. They work as secretaries, nurses, teachers, and store clerks, but also as electricians, construction workers, and telephone installers. It no longer makes sense for women to spend long hours at work and yet be expected to please everyone at home, too.

As a woman, you have a right to be your own person. Family life should be everybody's job, not just yours. Your mate does not have the right to hit you if dinner is not on the table when expected or to think that housework and child care are "women's work." Do not continue to do everything yourself and feel angry inside. Speak up; you will never get help if you do not ask for it.

Of course, if you have small children there are things you *must* do to care for them. They are unable to take care of themselves and depend on you to do it. While they are small, you can *never* leave them unsupervised, even for just a few minutes. You will have little time for yourself, and there will be days when you are totally "fed up" with taking care of children. As soon as they are older, try to teach them to do things for themselves so that they will learn that mothers have rights, too.

What things do you do to please others? . . . Are you easily talked into going places and doing things because other people want to—even though you would rather not? . . . If someone gives you a few cents less than the right change at a store, do you ask for what you did not get? . . . If you try on several pairs of shoes at a store, do you feel you have to buy at least one pair? . . . Do you jump up to wait on your mate or children whenever they want something? . . . Does your family know how to make you feel guilty? . . . These are the kinds of things you can change. You can learn to be assertive and tell other people what *you* want and need and not continue to live your life as a second-class citizen.

PASSIVE BEHAVIOR

If you behave passively, you do not say what you really mean or tell people how you feel. You let others take advantage of you. You do what you are told, even if inside you do not really want to. You may feel mad at others or yourself. You may cry or only hint at what you want and expect others to read your mind. If you try to please everyone else, avoid fighting or arguing, or give in so people will like you, you are being passive.

When You Act Passively, You:

Never say what you really want; others have to guess what it is

Say "I'm sorry" and "I guess" too much

Let other people tell you what to do and how you feel

Do not speak up for yourself

May feel tense or shaky

Look down and do not look others in the eye

Walk like a victim, not a powerful person

AGGRESSIVE BEHAVIOR

If you are aggressive, you tell others how you really think or feel about something, but you make other people angry because of your attitude. You blame and threaten them, point or shake your finger at them, yell insults, and demand what you want *now*. You may even fight to get your own way. Maybe you *will* get what you want, but you will not feel good about it, and neither will others.

When You Act Aggressively, You:

Blame others with "you" statements
Look angry, threaten others, or shake your finger at them
Are usually loud, may yell, and insist on what you want "right now"
Accuse others and tell them what they "need" to do

"You" Statements Blame Others:

You made me—; You always—; You never—; You charged me too much—; You got my order wrong—.

ASSERTIVE BEHAVIOR

If you are an assertive person, you express your true thoughts and feelings in ways that do not hurt others. You say what you really want or need and are willing to stand up for yourself, but you do not run over people to do so. You think about what other people need and want, too, and try to work things out without making them mad. You feel relaxed and good about yourself.

When You Act Assertively, You:

Use "I" statements
Say what you really want, feel, or think
Do not say things to hurt other people
Are reasonable
Listen to the other person
Use a pleasant voice and look at them

"I" Messages Tell Others How You Feel:

I feel angry when you—; I get upset when—; I think you may have made a mistake—; I have been waiting a long time—.

IF YOU ARE PASSIVE, YOU FEEL:

Hurt, unhappy, and mad at yourself.

IF YOU ARE AGGRESSIVE, YOU FEEL:

Better than others, "right," angry, on edge, as if others
are trying to take advantage of you.

IF YOU ARE ASSERTIVE, YOU FEEL:

Relaxed, honest, as if you deserve respect, in charge
of your life.

WHEN YOU ARE PASSIVE, OTHERS FEEL:

Angry with you because they are not sure what you
want, better than you are.

WHEN YOU ARE AGGRESSIVE, OTHERS FEEL:

Hurt, angry, as if they have to protect themselves from
your attack, insulted or "put down."

WHEN YOU ARE ASSERTIVE, OTHERS FEEL:

That you are being reasonable,
that you understand their point of view,
that you can work out an agreement.

IF YOU ARE PASSIVE:

You want everyone to like you.
You want to please everyone.

But instead:

You hardly ever get what you want.
Other people take advantage of you.
You feel angry inside but are afraid to show it outside.
You may take that anger out on others.
You may have headaches or other physical symptoms.
You feel lonely and isolated.

IF YOU ARE AGGRESSIVE:

You want to be in power.
You want to put others down.
You want to frighten others into doing what you want.

But instead:

You may get what you want, but you have to hurt others to get it.
People want to "get even" with you.
You do not respect the rights of others.
You feel "uptight."
Others do not like or respect you.

IF YOU ARE ASSERTIVE:

You want to express your true feelings, wants,
   and needs.
You respect others and want them to respect you.

And what happens is:

You usually get what you want, if is within reason.
You feel good about yourself.
You respect the rights of others.
You can work out an agreement that is good for both
   sides.

ROLE-PLAYS: WHAT DO YOU DO?

Role-play #1: You are in a restaurant and the service is terrible. You had to wait almost an hour for your food, and it is cold when you get it. How do you handle it?

- If you are passive? . . . (Do not say anything, and maybe do not leave a tip so they will know you were unhappy.)
- If you are aggressive? . . . (Scream at the waitress, tell her what you think of her and the service, and cause a scene.)
- If you are assertive? . . . (Calmly tell the cashier when you leave that you were very displeased with the service and explain why, and maybe they will make an adjustment in your bill.)

Role-play #2: You are at a resource agency office. They tell you the paperwork you brought is not complete. You have to complete it before they can see you, so today's appointment is canceled. How do you handle it?

- If you are passive? . . . (You hang your head and leave without trying to explain why.)
- If you are aggressive? . . . (You scream, make a scene, threaten the worker.)
- If you are assertive? . . . (You explain that you have applied for the needed document, but it is not back yet. Ask if you can see the worker to tell her that.)

Role-play #3: Your friend calls on the phone and tells you about a problem she has been having. You have to leave to pick up your children at school. How do you handle it?

- If you are passive? . . . (You keep listening, while you get more and more upset about being late to pick up your children; you finally make up an excuse to get off the phone.)

- If you are aggressive? . . . (You say, "Why do you always have to dump on me? I have things to do, and I am too busy to listen to you.")
- If you are assertive? . . . (You say, "I have to go pick up the children at school, but call me back in thirty minutes, and we can talk then.")

Week Four: My Appearance

This week you will learn that how you look affects how you feel about yourself. If you are clean and neatly dressed, you will feel much better than if you are dressed in dirty clothing that needs repair.

General good habits, bathing, washing your hair, brushing your teeth, can affect not only how you look, but your health as well.

Even the colors you wear can brighten your appearance or make you look pale and tired. You will learn a little bit about makeup and hair care.

Listen carefully and you will be *looking good!*

AFFIRMATION

I choose to look good, to be clean and well-groomed, not just for others, but for myself.

I will keep my clothing washed and in good repair, even if that is sometimes hard to do.

I will learn as much as I can about how I can improve my appearance.

I will practice what I learn with my family.

Week Five:
My Time for Myself

We all need a "break" sometimes—time to do what we really want to do for ourselves. Today you will have an opportunity to express your emotions and also to create something pretty and useful. You may have never tried to do any craft before, but you *can* do it and do it well.

AFFIRMATION

I can allow myself to be different from everyone else and still be okay.

I can have feelings and be warm and kind.

I can allow myself to like me as I am.

I can do "fun" things because I want to, without a reason.

I will allow myself to do what *I* want to do, just for *me*, because I deserve it.

I will make time every day to do at least one nice thing for myself, not always for others.

Allowing myself to be happy makes me feel better about myself.

JUST BE YOU

It is okay to be different. You do not have to be just like your mother, or your father, or anyone else in your family. You do not have to be what other people want you to be; you can just be you. Being different is what makes other people want to know you and like you.

Can you imagine how dull it would be if everyone were just alike? Everyone would have the same color hair and eyes and would look the same. When a baby was born, nobody would have to wonder what it would look like; they would already know. All the houses and cars would look alike; even all of the business buildings would look alike because everyone would like the same things. Nobody would be tall or short, or fat or thin. Nobody would be sad or happy, or funny or grouchy. That would be a terrible world.

It is all right to make mistakes or to forget things. That is part of being human, and no humans are perfect. It is better to make a mistake than not to try at all. You can change your mind if you want to and change your whole life if you choose to. You can take time every day to do something for yourself, not always for others. You can take time to be happy, to laugh, to sing, and to enjoy being alive.

Learn to enjoy just being *you*!

Week Six: My Friends

Do you know how to be a friend, or how to keep a friend, or even how to *make* friends? You have to treat friends the way you would want them to treat you, or they will not be around for long.

This week you will explore friendship from every side, and discover what you do right or wrong in your relationships.

AFFIRMATION

I will learn to love myself.
I am a worthwhile person.
I deserve to be happy.
I do not have to please everyone.
I deserve to be loved and respected by others.
I will choose friends that make me feel good about myself.

PUTTY PEOPLE

Are you a "putty person," one who shapes yourself exactly as someone else wants you to? Do you want so much to be liked that you give up what *you* want for what *others* want? Do you pretend you have no likes or dislikes of your own, no opinions of your own, and bend yourself all out of shape to be the person someone else wants you to be?

Putty people never make their own decisions; they wait for someone else to tell them what to decide. They never tell anyone else where they want to eat, what movie they want to see, or what they want to do on the weekend.

The worst thing about being a putty person is that you change yourself into the shape someone else wants you to be, and you forget what you looked like to begin with. Pretty soon you are no longer yourself at all; you are squeezed into a new and different shape, and you have no memory of what you used to be.

Do not let others make you a putty person; stand up for yourself; express yourself and be the kind of special person that makes other people want *your* opinion.

HOW TO BE A FRIEND

Show respect and consideration for others.

If other people always take advantage of you, ask yourself how you are acting to make them treat you that way. Maybe *you* have to change.

Do not scream at people to make them do what you want; it does not work.

Tell other people when they do a good job, and tell them why you believe in them.

You do not have to agree with everything someone says to be his or her friend. Differences make people more interesting.

Ask questions before you accept gossip; what you heard may not be true.

Do not tell people things for "their own good." This often hurts feelings.

Do not complain about your life or about things you cannot control.

Be dependable; do what you say you will do.

Do not be afraid to admit you are wrong.

Do not be afraid to care about others, be there for them, or listen to them.

Get other people's opinions, but make up your own mind. You do not need permission to live your own life.

Be an example; do not just tell others what to do.

Reach out to meet new people; do not always wait for them to make the first move.

True friends are not made overnight. Anyone who wants to be your best friend immediately may have something else in mind.

Remember, only *you* can make yourself happy; nobody else can do it for you.

People usually do not give a lot of thought to what they want from their friends. Why do you consider someone your friend? Is she helpful, caring, dependable, and always there when you are down? Can you have the same relationship with everyone—your boss, your doctor, or the cashier at the grocery store? Probably you cannot; all of our friendships are different because we want different things from different people.

Do not expect your friends to be perfect. They may let you down, just as you may let them down sometimes. They may have had a bad day or said something that hurt your feelings without meaning to. Expect the best, but do not give up on them if they fall short once in a while. Talk it out; do not go away mad.

What you want out of a friendship may not be the same as what your friend wants. Find out what she wants from you, as well as what you want from her. Do not expect your friend to be with you every minute, and especially—do not expect her to be your *only* friend. Being jealous of her time and attention can break up your friendship. You need other friends just as she does.

It is great to have friends to share your troubles, your joys, and just to talk with. But there are limits. Do you say hurtful things and insult them? Just because someone is your friend does not give you the right to tell her all her faults, tell her she looks terrible, or hurt her in any way. Saying that you did not mean it does not make her feel better.

Do you take advantage of your friends, always taking from them and never giving to them? Most people do not mind helping you out sometimes, but if you want a friend to take you to the grocery store one day, downtown the next, and to a doctor appointment the next, she may begin to feel you only want her for a friend because she has a car.

Do you ask a friend to take care of your children for "just a little while" and not come back for hours? Do that several times, and your friend will refuse to help you at all. Do you borrow from her constantly, so that she says to herself, "Oh, no . . . here she comes again!" when she sees you coming to the door?

In order to have friends you must realize that they have lives, too. Treat them the way you would like to be treated.

Week Seven: My Education

Did you know that you do not have to finish high school or have a GED to get into some colleges? Did you know that women who are reentering the job market may be able to get tuition assistance from a government agency? Did you know that there are many grants, scholarships, and other programs that can help pay all or part of your college tuition? Did you know that the government, along with local agencies, sponsors many job-training programs?

If you want to finish high school, go to college, or get job training, there are many opportunities available. You will hear about all of this and more during this session.

AFFIRMATION

I am a worthwhile person.
I can do anything I want to do.
I can choose to finish school or get more training to get a job, if that is what I want to do.
I will live my life for myself, not always just for others.
I will learn who I am and work to become the best person I can be.

MONEY

O money, money, money,
   I am not necessarily one of those
   who think thee holy.

But I often stop to wonder
How thou canst go out so fast
When thou comest in so slowly.

—Ogden Nash

IN CHARGE

You are in charge of your life.
No matter what happens to you,
there are always many things that you control.

You have to decide what you want,
how badly you want it,
and how you will go about getting it.

Set reasonable goals;
work on those goals one at a time,
and you can make your dreams
become reality.

EXCUSES

I cannot be a success because:
   My family was poor.
   I have little education.
   I have physical limitations.
   I am too young.
   The job market is poor.
   I am too old.
   I have too many children.
   My mate will not want me to.
   I am afraid to get out of my present situation.
   I owe too many bills.
   I am too thin.
   I do not have enough money.
   I am not smart enough.

I am too fat.
I do not have a job.
Nobody likes me.
I live in a bad neighborhood.
I do not have a car.
What excuses have *you* used?

WHAT THINGS CAN I DO WELL?

I like working with my hands and fixing things that break down. I like to build things and use tools. I like to take things apart or put them together. I will be happiest in a job that lets me touch things or make things with my hands or run a machine.

I am good at typing, keeping things in order, solving problems, and having set times to do things. I like to work with numbers and details. I will be happiest in a job that is organized, perhaps working with computers or numbers or in an office.

I am good at using things in new ways. I like to talk to people and find out things about them. I think in words or pictures and like to write things down. I will be happiest in a job that lets me do things my own way and express my feelings. I like to do things when I want to, not when I have to. I may want to be involved with music, drawing, painting, or writing. I may want to invent new things or find new ways to use old ones.

I enjoy talking to people and getting them to do things or buy things. I like to work with other people, not by myself. I like to help people or teach them. I will be happiest in a job selling things or working in a store or restaurant. I would be a good nurse, doctor, teacher, social worker, or person who helps others do something.

DO YOU WANT A JOB?

When you *really* need a job for money to just *survive* from day to day you cannot be choosy. Many jobs are not exactly what you want, and they may not be ones you want to keep for the rest of your life but may be okay for a little while. Do your best there, but keep looking for something else. Remember, your goal is a job you can do, one you like, and one that makes you feel good about yourself.

Many jobs only require reading, writing, simple math, the ability to follow directions, talk to people, and learn new things from someone who shows you what to do. You may also need to know how to drive a car. You can probably do most of those things now and find something to support yourself on your way to your *goal* job.

Choose your goal job; write down what it is and all of the steps you have to take to reach it. Do not choose something you know is impossible to reach, rather something you feel you can really do. How can you take those steps? You may need to get your GED, go to junior college, university, trade school, or get on-the-job training to learn new skills. Take one step at a time and have faith in your ability to reach your goal. It may take a while, but if you keep climbing the ladder, you will eventually reach the top. Then you will be prepared to get your goal job—the job you have always wanted!

Week Eight: My Health

This week, you will learn how to protect yourself from illness, as well as how to keep yourself healthy from day to day. We will discuss risks you can control, as well as ones you cannot. If you do not now get a yearly physical exam, we will tell you why you should. If your lifestyle includes drugs and unsafe sex, you will learn the risks of that behavior. If you never learned the basics of how your body works, we will cover that also. If you have questions you never felt you could ask, this is the time to ask them, and we will try to give you answers.

AFFIRMATION

I choose to do everything I can to stay healthy.

I deserve to take care of my own health as well as that of my family.

I will learn all I can about my body and how to protect myself from illness.

I will seek medical care when I need it and not wait for things to "go away."

I will learn to relax and take things easier, without getting stressed over little things.

THINGS I CANNOT CHANGE ABOUT MY HEALTH

My sex—each sex gets different illnesses.

My race—some races are more susceptible to high blood pressure, some to diabetes, etc.

My age—you are always getting older; you cannot make yourself younger.

Who my parents and grandparents were—heredity may make it more likely that you will get certain illnesses or that you may live a long, healthy life.

What other things can you think of?

THINGS I CAN *CHANGE*

My diet, by eating healthy food

Getting more exercise

Quitting smoking or drinking too much

Not taking drugs or having unsafe sex

Having a yearly physical exam by a doctor or clinic

Having tests to be sure I do not have cancer, such as pap smears and mammograms when I am over forty

What other things can you think of?

Week Nine: My Family

If your family gave you more "Spears" than "Cheers," you probably grew up with lots of holes in your self-image. People often say things to children that hurt even though they may not really mean them.

It takes courage to change. It takes courage to think about yourself in new ways, to forget what you heard, and to remember that it is not true now, and in fact, it may *never* have been true.

Things that happened to you as a child affect how you feel today. You may feel guilty; you may never express your anger; you may "stuff" your feelings down inside and pretend that things do not bother you. You may feel that you do not deserve to have good things happen to you because you are a "bad" person and should be punished.

Do not blame others for everything. Quit using excuses that keep you in the same old rut. You are responsible for your own life, and you *can* make things better.

If you were treated badly as a child, it will be harder for you to treat your own children in better ways. If you were never shown love, it will be harder for you to show it to others. If your house was always dirty, it will be harder for you to keep yours clean now. If your parents did not care if you were at home instead of in trouble, it will be harder for you to control your own children.

All of these things may make you feel depressed, as if you are crying on the inside, or they may make you confused about what is happening in your family now. They may make you feel that you are a bad person or a bad parent. Just because these things happened to you in the past, or even if they are happening now, it does not mean that your future is hopeless. You *can* learn new ways, and it can be the beginning of something better for all of you.

No matter how bad you feel about yourself, or how bad you think you are, *nobody* has the right to hit you, no matter what you do or say. It is not your fault, no matter how many times you are told that it is. Telling you "I'm sorry" does *not* make it OK. If you or your children are in danger, get out *immediately.* Call a friend, your family, the police, a shelter, but get out of the house *right then!*

AFFIRMATION

I choose to do everything I can to make my family a happy one.

I will remember IALAC, and I will not let others destroy me with "poison" statements.

I will remember that what my parents or others told me when I was small may not have been true.

I will think in "Cheers," not in "Spears."

Week Ten:
My Financial Responsibility

This is a subject everyone is interested in. How to spend your money wisely, and how to get the most for what you have to spend is something we all need to learn. You are going to learn how to make your money last all month, as well as how to shop "smart." Shopping for groceries can be easy, but there are some secrets you may not have learned. Your local grocery store is not going to tell you how to save money, but we are.

AFFIRMATION

I will learn to budget my money so it will cover my expenses for the month.
I choose to pay all my bills and to be sure they are paid on time.
I choose to be a careful shopper and get the most I can for my money.
I will prepare sensible meals and not eat only "junk food."
I will learn to have a positive attitude even when things are difficult for me.

YOUR MONEY AND HOW TO MANAGE IT

Basic budgeting can be done by dividing money for bills into separate envelopes. That way you can be sure all bills are paid before the money is spent on something else. You can also tell if you will have extra money to spend on something you want or need. Sometimes emergencies come up, and you will not have enough money to pay all of your bills. You need to know about places you can go to get help. Many churches have programs that help with food and clothing, and there are usually agencies in your area that help with things such as rent and utilities. Sometimes those agencies run out of money, just like you do, and they may not be able to help you when you need help. If you cannot get the money, or anything else you need, explain the situation to the people you owe; do not just hope the problem will go away. It will only get worse if you ignore it.

SMART SHOPPING

Try to shop in large, chain grocery stores or warehouse-type stores in suburban areas if at all possible. These usually have lower prices than stores in poorer neighborhoods. The store owners know that if you are unable to leave the area you will have to pay whatever they charge. They also say that they have to raise prices due to stealing and having more security needs. The very worst places to shop are small convenience stores; they will charge as much as they can get away with just because they know you are close by. They may offer to give you credit, but you are paying dearly for it.

Know how to shop. Read labels. They tell you what is in the products and how much per unit or ounce. The first ingredient listed on the label is the one contained in the highest quantity, and they continue in order, most to least, downward. Labels tell you how many calories and how much fat products contain, as well as other information.

Compare sizes and prices. The large economy or family size may not be the cheapest; the smaller size may be on sale, or the price may be the same for the same number of ounces. If you have to throw out part of a product because it is too large to use up, it is not a bargain; you will do better to buy a smaller size even if it costs a little more. Read shelf labels and compare products; one may be on sale, or one brand may always cost less.

Use generic products (ones without brand names) or store brands. Many of them cost much less than brand-name products; some cost *half* the price. You may not feel their quality is as good but at least try them. Most of them are made by the same large manufacturers but are labeled with the store brand and sold for less money. Brand-name products cost more in order to pay for advertising.

Use coupons. Manufacturers and local stores are giving you money to try their products, hoping that you will like them and continue to buy them. Stores that offer double or triple the money for coupons are charging you more for other things in their stores, otherwise they would be losing money. Grocery stores make very little profit, but some are cheaper than others. Compare the stores in your area, and shop in the one that best suits your needs.

Cook things from "scratch." You are paying for every step the food manufacturer takes to save you time. Unless you feel the time you save is worth the money (when you have to fix a quick meal) always buy foods separately and mix them yourself. If you buy one of the "helpers," you are paying almost double what the separate ingredients cost.

Buy "stretchers." Those are rice, beans, macaroni, spaghetti, and noodles. They can be mixed with hamburger, leftover meats, sauces, soups, and seasonings to make one-dish meals for very little money.

Try to shop no more than once a week, less often if possible. This will help keep your food bill down, as every trip to the store adds to the temptation to buy expensive or junk foods you do not really need.

Make out menus. Plan your meals for the week around products you see on sale in grocery store ads. Know before you go to the store what things you need for the week. Do not go to the store when you are hungry; you will buy everything you see and a lot you do not need. Leave your kids with someone if you can; if they do not see it, they cannot want it!

Shop for staples (products you need to cook, such as flour, sugar, salt, and oil) early in the month. Get peanut butter, canned foods, the "stretchers" already mentioned, and things that keep without refrigeration then, too. Buy milk, eggs, bread, dairy products, and other perishables to "fill-in" as needed during the month.

Watch for seasonal specials. Buy certain foods in season. Do not buy watermelon in December. Stock up on picnic foods near Fourth of July. Buy turkey in November and December. Go to the farmer's market in the summertime to get fresh vegetables and fruits.

Try to feed your family a healthy diet, not just junk food. Make sure you choose foods from all of the food groups so your children will have the building blocks they need to grow up strong and in good health.

Look for bargains in other things as well as groceries. Do not forget garage sales, resale shops, flea markets, and Goodwill and Salvation Army stores. Look for end-of-season sales at department and discount stores; go to close-out, outlet, and off-price stores. Trade your children's outgrown clothing with a friend. Watch for shoe sales, as shoes can seldom be handed down.

Week Eleven:
My Homemaking Skills

If you have never thought about how important food is to how you look and feel, you will after this three-week series.

Did you know that breakfast is one of the most important meals in your day? Do you know how much, and what, you should feed a small child? Do you think you have to have at least one serving of meat every day? Do you think children should drink as much milk as they want at every meal?

You will learn the answers to these questions and many more during this week and the following two weeks. When you have finished the series, your family will be on its way to a healthier diet.

AFFIRMATION

I am a creative and worthwhile person even though I make mistakes.

I will take care of my family's health and well-being and make my home a happy, comfortable place.

I will learn to say "I can" even when my fear wants me to say "I cannot."

I will remember that I have the power to change my life.

FINISH EVERY DAY

Finish every day and be done with it.
You have done what you could.

Some mistakes may have been made;
Forget them as soon as you can.

Tomorrow is a new day.
Begin it with peace and happiness and feeling too well to worry
   about yesterday.

This day is good, with its own hopes and joys, and it is too rich a
   gift to waste a moment on yesterdays.

—paraphrased from a poem by
Ralph Waldo Emerson

Week Twelve:
Second Week, Homemaking

AFFIRMATION

I am okay as I am; I do not have to be perfect.
I will learn to love myself, as I cannot learn to love others unless
  I do.
I will learn as much as I can so that I can help myself and others.
I am in control of my own life.

FAMILY RULES

> If you sleep in it—make it up.
> If you wear it—hang it up.
> If you eat out of it—put it in the sink.
> If you step on it—wipe it off.
> If you open it—close it.
> If you empty it—fill it up.
> If it rings—answer it.
> If it howls—feed it.
> If it cries—love it.

> > –original author unknown

SPICE LIST

You are going to use this list to write down which spices you can identify from what they look and smell like. Numbered samples of different spices will be passed around the group, and you will write the number in front of the spice you think it matches.

Chili powder ____
Vanilla ____
Green pepper ____
Cinnamon ____
Black pepper ____
Allspice ____
Poultry seasoning ____
Celery seed ____
Oregano ____
Basil ____
Sage ____
Garlic salt or powder ____
Cloves ____
Dill ____
Onion salt or powder ____
Nutmeg ____

You may want to take notes on what foods to season with which spices. Learn to use more than just salt and pepper!

Week Thirteen:
Third Week, Homemaking

AFFIRMATION

I am not perfect, as nobody is perfect.
I will do my best and be the best person I can be.
I will love myself as I am and not feel I always fall short and
   need changing.
I will learn all I can in order to take care of myself and my
   family.

You may want to make notes here on what you learn today.
You may also have decided to collect recipes from your group
and put them in a special folder or booklet. If you have a kitchen
available where you have your class, you may be able to cook
meals that are low cost, good for you, and delicious. If so, you
can eat those during the break or at the end of the session.

Week Fourteen: My Goals

You are going to be learning how to set goals and how to reach the ones you set. It is a simple process, but it takes lots of work. The first step is to decide what you really want for yourself and believe that you can reach your goal. You have to consider your limitations; if you are thirty-five and have four children, you likely will not want to study law because it will take too long. If you faint at the sight of blood, you probably would not make a good nurse. If you have severe asthma, you might get sick from selling perfume.

Decide whether you need help to reach your goal; will you need a babysitter or help from someone else? Your goal may not be to get a job; it may be to treat your child better or to move to a new apartment. Whatever it is, you might not be able to reach your goal alone. Be sure you ask the "other" person if they are willing to help you reach it.

Write down what you want to do. Plan all of the small steps it will take to make your dream come true. Put them in order, starting with whichever comes first. Do not say, "I will do either this—or that." You will never reach your goal if you cannot decide what you really want for yourself.

Now, start with the first step, and keep taking steps until you come to the end of the list. Remember, it will take time and lots of hard work, but you *can* do it!

AFFIRMATION

I am all right as I am even though I am not perfect.

Mistakes are things I wish I had done differently or things I did not do that I wish I had done.

I will learn from my mistakes so I will not make the same ones over and over.

I will forgive myself for the mistakes I have made and go on with my life.

I will set new goals and not be discouraged by past failures.

I will believe in myself.

CHANGING

Think about your life the way it is today. If you want it to be different, you must believe that *you* are the one who can change it. Life does not just "happen" to you; you *make* it happen.

> Nobody can *stop* you from changing your life.
> Nobody can *make* you change your life.

> Only you know how you want to change it.
> You have to begin and change it step by step.

WINNERS AND LOSERS

Do you think you are a winner? Winners follow through on what they say they will do. Losers only make promises. Winners listen. Losers just wait until it is their turn to talk. Winners do more than their job. Losers say "I only work here." Winners respect those who know more than they do and try to learn from them. Losers try to show them up for what they do not know. In LAMS you are learning to be a winner. Saying good things to yourself, and learning to believe them, can make you a winner.

We begin every LAMS session with a positive affirmation—something that makes you feel better about yourself. You should repeat such affirmations to yourself every day. Write them on a piece of paper and put them on the bathroom mirror or on the refrigerator door—anyplace where you will see them many times during the day. When you believe you are a good person and in control of your life, you can plan ahead and set goals. Your thinking changes from believing you can do nothing to realizing that you can do almost anything. What you tell yourself can change your life.

Week Fifteen: Celebration

This session is a time to have fun; something you forget to do sometimes. Everyone deserves to have a good time, to play, and to remember what it is like to be a child. The child you used to be is still there, grown older, but not gone entirely, so enjoy!

AFFIRMATION

I am a good person.

I am a happy person.

I can do anything I set my mind to, if I really work hard.

There are some things I cannot change; I will learn to accept these things.

I have a right to enjoy myself and others around me, to laugh and play.

THE LAMS PROGRAM
FOR CHANGING YOUR LIFE

You learn many things in LAMS. If you are at or near completion of the course, you will remember many of the lessons and hopefully are practicing them. If you have just begun to attend, you have many sessions ahead of you that will give you a blueprint for changing your life. Positive affirmations, or things that make you feel good about yourself, should become a part of your thinking every day. What you think determines how you feel. Learning to make choices, set goals, and get along with others are all important parts of the LAMS program. You have learned, or will learn, that what you heard as a child is not necessarily true today and, in fact, may not have been true then. Education, good health, sensible shopping, and proper nutrition are all keys to living the kind of life you want to live. Good luck in shaping that new life!

Recommended Readings for Parents

Baer, Jean (1976). *How to Be an Assertive (Not Aggressive) Woman in Life, in Love, and on the Job.* New York: Penguin Books USA, Inc.

Branden, Nathaniel (1983). *Honoring the Self.* New York: Bantam Books.

Burns, David, MD (1985). *Intimate Connections.* New York: Signet.

Capacchione, Lucia (1982). *The Creative Journal for Children.* Boston, MA: Shambhala.

Carpenter, Zerle L., Director Texas Agricultural Extension Service (1990). *Eating Right is Basic* and other publications. Austin, TX: Texas Agricultural Service.

Carter, Steve (1990) *What Smart Women Know.* New York: M. Evans.

Clarke, Jean Illsley (1978). *Self-Esteem: A Family Affair.* California: Harper & Row.

Cole-Whittaker, Terry (1989). *Love and Power in a World Without Limits.* New York: Harper & Row.

Drakeford, John W. (1976). *Do Your Hear Me, Honey?* New York: Harper & Row.

Fluegelman, Andrew (1981). *More New Games.* Berkeley, CA: Headlands Press.

Forward, Dr. Susan (1989). *Toxic Parents.* New York: Bantam Books.

Hendricks, Gay, PhD (1990). *Learning to Love Yourself Workbook.* New York: Prentice Hall.

John-Roger and Peter McWilliams (1991). *Life 101.* Los Angeles, CA: Prelude Press.

Johnson, Barbara (1990). *Pain Is Inevitable but Misery Is Optional.* Dallas, TX: Word Publishing.

Johnson, Barbara (1992). *Splashes of Joy in the Cesspools of Life.* Dallas, TX: Word Publishing.

Johnson, Barbara (1993). *Pack Up Your Gloomees in a Great Big Box, Then Sit on the Lid and Laugh!* Dallas, TX: Word Publishing.

Kagan, Richard and Shirley Schlosberg (1989). *Families in Perpetual Crisis.* New York: W. W. Norton and Company, Inc.

Leman, Kevin (1987). *The Pleasers, Women Who Can't Say NO—and the Men Who Control Them.* New York: Dell Publishing.

Lennox, Joan Hatch and Judith Hatch Shapiro (1990). *Lifechanges.* New York: Crown Publishers, Inc.

Marone, Nicky (1992). *Women and Risk.* New York: St. Martin's Press.

Matthews, Andrew (1988). *Being Happy.* California: Price Stern Sloan, Inc.

Matthews, Andrew (1991). *Making Friends.* California: Price Stern Sloan, Inc.

McKay, Matthew, PhD, and Patrick Fanning (1987). *Self-Esteem.* Oakland, CA: Harbinger.

Miller, Keith, and Andrea Wells Miller (1981). *The Single Experience*. Dallas, TX: Word Publishing.

Palmer, Pat, EdD (1977). *Liking Myself*. San Luis Obispo, CA: Impact Publishers.

Paul, Jordan, PhD, and Margaret Paul, PhD (1987). *If You Really Loved Me*. Minneapolis, MN: CompCare Publishers

Phelps, Stanlee, and Nancy Austin (1985). *The Assertive Woman*. San Luis Obispo, CA: Impact Publishers.

Pilkington, Maya, and the Diagram Group (1987). *The Real Life Aptitude Test*. New York: Pharos Books.

Semigran, Candace (1988). *One Minute Self Esteem—Caring for Yourself and Others*. New York: Bantam Books.

Sheperd, Scott, PhD (1990). *What Do You Think of YOU?* Minneapolis, MN: CompCare Publishers.

Sherman, Robert, and Norman Fredman (1986). *Handbook of Structured Techniques in Marriage and Family Therapy*. New York: Brunner/Mazel, Inc.

Texas Department of Human Services. *Assertiveness for Neglecting Mothers*. Austin, TX: TDHS.

Thoele, Sue Patton (1988). *The Courage to Be Yourself*. Nevada City, CA: Pyramid Press.

Viscott, David (1977). *Risking*. New York: Simon and Schuster.

Woititz, Janet G., EdD (1992). *Healthy Parenting*. New York: Simon and Schuster/Fireside.